# Natural Cures

## *20 Natural Cures, Herbal Medicines, And Natural Remedies For Increased Overall Health And Beauty!*

I0419839

**Sarah Brooks**

# STOP!!! Before you read any further....Would you like to know the secrets of Anti Aging?

If your answer is yes, then you are not alone. Thousands of people are looking for the secret to reducing wrinkles, looking younger, and maintaining a youthful appearance.

If you have been searching for these answers without much luck, you are in the right place!

Not only will you gain incredible insight in this book, but because I want to make sure to give you as much value as possible, right now for a limited time you can get full **100% FREE access to a VIP bonus Ebook** entitled **Anti Aging Made Easy!**

## Just Go Here For Free Instant Access:

## www.LuxyLifeNaturals.com

# Legal Notice

# Disclaimer Notice

# Table Of Contents

# Introduction

I want to thank you and congratulate you for purchasing the book, *Natural Cures: 20 Natural Cures, Herbal Medicines, And Natural Remedies For Increased Overall Health And Beauty!*

This "Natural Cures" book contains proven steps and strategies on how to make use of what's available in your pantry and garden when it comes to treating common ailments.

There are countless benefits to going natural with your medication. Aside from the fact that natural cures are readily available, they are also known to be less toxic to our bodies. This is especially important if you intend on using them continuously.

In this book, you'll learn more about:

*1. Benefits Of Natural Cures*

*2. 20 Natural Cures To Heal The Body*

*3. Herbal Medicines For Common Ailments In The Elderly*

*4. List Of Healing Foods*

*5. Using Essential Oils For Natural Cures*

*6. Why Natural Cures Vs. Traditional Medications*

*7. Natural Cures For Migraines And Headaches*

*8. Natural Cures For Skin Diseases And Acne*

*9. Natural Cures For Arthritis*

*10. Natural Cures For High Blood Pressure*

We hope you find the content useful and that you give it a try for yourself in order to really experience its benefits.

Thanks again for purchasing this book, I hope you enjoy it!

# Chapter 1: Benefits Of Natural Cures

There are a lot of great things often said about the use of natural cures when it comes to treating certain ailments; from the most common to some of the more advanced diseases, there always seem to be a homeopathic remedy meant just for it. However, there are still those who are more on the skeptical side of things. After all, modern medicine works just fine, so why should they change to something that's mostly untested?

The answer is quite simple. Homeopathic therapy, or natural cures, takes into consideration the overall health of the individual while curing them of what's ailing their bodies. This is something that modern medications tend to overlook and in some way, people are often told to prepare themselves for the possible side-effects of a particular medicine. If you think about it, this is like curing a sickness in exchange for a less deadly one-- but a sickness nonetheless. Can that be called a cure? For some, it is no more than a band-aid approach to getting better.

To help you understand things better, let's take a closer look at the benefits of using natural cures and therapies.

1. *Cleaner and safer.* Because it uses raw materials that are also often found in your food, you can rest assured that it is fine for your body to ingest it. You may not know it, but many of the herbs that you consume on a daily basis have positive effects on your body-- and when combined with other plants that compliment it? The effects only get better and more potent.

1. *More affordable.* It is no secret that manufactured medicines can easily burn through an average person's savings. This is also one of the reasons why some people would rather not treat their illnesses as they don't have the finances to do so. Luckily for them, there is a cheaper alternative. Because the ingredients needed for it are

readily available, they are far more affordable. You can even do it yourself, right in the comfort of your own home using materials straight out of the pantry.

- *You can grow them yourself.* In doing so, you're also able to save even more money and perhaps, make money on the side if you decide to sell some of what you're able to grow. Medicinal plants and herbs are quite easy to plant and maintain, all you need is the right knowledge to do so. The next time you get sick, you're walking to your garden instead of to the pharmacy.

- *Milder.* Manufactured medicines can be harsh to the body; we've already pointed this out. They have certain ingredients that can actually cause damage with prolonged use. In fact, some of them can even affect the healthy cells in the body and cause a weaker immune system. On the other hand, all natural cures target the problem specifically while aiding our body in fighting any infection. In fact, there are known natural remedies which can boost the immune system all while treating the problem.

- *They can often be used in conjunction with modern medicine for an even more potent treatment to the ailments that you have.* Though not all doctors agree with it, there are those who will allow their patients to take herbal supplements as long as it complements the treatments they are currently receiving.

# Chapter 2: 20 Natural Cures To Heal The Body

At any given time, your entire body can throw you for a loop. Waking up with a sore throat that seemingly came out of nowhere or a great lunch that leaves you with an indigestion. Maybe you overdid it with the exercising and your muscles have been aching so much that doing small things becomes a painful chore. Before you reach for a bottle of your usual medicine, stop and contemplate the possible effects for a minute. There are a lot of natural home remedies that can be put together by simply mixing a few different ingredients from your pantry. With these around, you won't even need to run to your local pharmacy.

So, shall we get started with learning more about them?

1. *Feeling nauseated?* First, infuse some fresh ginger with hot water. Strain it afterwards and freeze the liquid in ice cube trays. Once frozen, just consume the cubes the same way you would a candy. It's also great for people who are experiencing nausea due to pregnancy of after effects of surgery.

2. *Hiccups.* There is a quick natural solution for this! Just swallow a teaspoon or 2 of granulated sugar. It would effectively stimulate as well as reset the irritated nerve that's causing the spasms.

3. *Sore throats.* For this one, try some garlic. Gargling a solution of six pressed garlic cloves mixed with a glass of warm water would certainly help. Do this twice daily for the next 3 days and you'll be able to see and feel significant changes. This is all thanks to the very potent antimicrobial properties contained in garlic.

4. *Coughing.* Indulge yourself with a square or 2 of the dark chocolate as this contains more theobromine, a compound

that's far more effective than codeine when it comes to suppressing a cough. The best bit? It doesn't give you the same dizziness or the constipation.

5. *Night coughs.* Chocolate might make it harder for you to fall asleep at night so an alternative would be honey. 2 teaspoons for younger kids should work well and a tablespoon for adults should be enough to soothe both the coughing, and raw feeling in your throat which could be quite uncomfortable. You can also mix a bit of natural vitamin C supplement with it, 500mg should work for this purpose. The combination of the two helps in boosting the immune system, ridding you of the cough early on.

6. *Reducing a fever.* Linden flower tea, in particular, works in two different ways when it comes to helping you. First, it stimulates the hypothalamus so that it controls your temperature better. Next, it dilates your blood vessels which induces sweating. Just a tablespoon of the dried herb, steeped in hot water can be of great benefit. Drink it at least three times each day.

7. *Accidentally burn yourself?* A dab of aloe Vera would immediately soothe it and help your skin heal faster. It's anti-inflammatory properties also help reduce the redness and swelling while creating a kind of second skin, shielding any exposed nerve endings from the air around you. It's also a great looking plant to have at home!

8. *Flatulence.* We all get this every now and then and it can be quite uncomfortable. For this, some peppermint would be quite handy. The important bit to remember is how you should ingest it. Two enteric coated peppermint capsules, weighing about 500mg grams each should be enough.

9. *Treating colds.* For this, vitamin C is highly needed. Sipping on a faux hot toddy certainly helps. All you need to do is cut a lemon in half and squeeze the juice from it into a nice cup. Add some boiling water to this and a teaspoon of

some organic honey as well. Both immunity boosters that help in lessening the discomfort in your throat. Even the vapors from this mix helps so do inhale it to open up your sinuses. Two cups each day is highly recommended.

10. *Foot odor*? This could be caused by a variety of different things but there is one very effective natural remedy for it. Soak your feet in a mixture of 1 part vinegar and 2 parts water to eliminate any bacteria on it. You can also take a daily foot bath in strong black tea, just let it cool first.

11. *Bad breath*? A great solution for it would be gargling with some acidic lemon juice as it can effectively kill any odor causing bacteria in your mouth. Another method is to eat some plain yogurt which would also kill bad bacteria in your mouth.

12. *Chapped lips*. These could be due to a lot of different things. Changes in the season or even lack of hydration. It can also heal broken skin very quickly so you'll find that within a few days, your lips are looking nice and supple once more.

13. *Relieving a stiff neck*. A quick blast of hot and cold water against the area would help get the blood circulating properly again. Run some warm water over your neck for 20 seconds before switching to cold and doing it for 10 seconds. Doing so should help constrict blood flow. Repeat it at least three times before you get out of the shower.

14. *Sunburn*. If you have olive oil or coconut oil around then you have all that you need. Both are capable of soothing and healing broken skin effectively. Just apply it directly onto the area before gently massaging it into your skin. Repeat at least twice a day until the area is completely healed.

15. *Insomnia*. Beat insomnia, not by using prescription medicine, but through natural means. Before bedtime, eat

a handful of cherries which are rich in melatonin and helps regulate sleeping patterns.

16. *Puffy and red eyes.* Using some black tea bags under your eyes would help. Just dip it in warm water for a few minutes, allow to cool then press it onto your closed eyes gently. Leave it on for 10 minutes and let the tannins in your tea do their job.

17. *Healing scarred skin.* Using rose hip oil is well-known in the beauty community when it comes to reducing the appearance of scars. Just apply it onto the affected area at least twice a day and you should see a difference within the first week, depending on the extent of the scarring.

18. *Headaches.* One of the most common problems that people get every single day. For this, have some magnesium handy. 200 to 400mg of this should be more than enough to reduce muscle spasms and tension that often cause your head to throb.

19. *Feeling acidic after a huge meal?* Try some lemon for dessert. Just cut one in half and drink its juice. This should help return the balance in your stomach as well as ease the pain that comes with acidity.

20. *Relieve menstrual cramps.* Take ½ to a teaspoon of crampbark tincture every 2 hours on the days when you get the worst cramps. This quickly relaxes the muscles and prevents them from tensing up, effectively diminishing the pain that you feel as well.

# Chapter 3: Herbal Medicines For Common Ailments In The Elderly

More often than not, people tend to associate ill health with aging but this is not always the case. In living an active lifestyle and having a good diet, it is very possible to keep one's mental vitality and physical endurance. Of course, having the right supplements also adds to this as commercially available medications can certainly become detrimental to the elderly with continued use.

In this chapter, we'll look at natural remedies for many of the health issues that often come with old age.

- *Gout, rheumatism and arthritis.* For this, rosemary, white willow and devil's claw will certainly help.

- *Brittle bones.* This is fairly common for people who reach a certain age and to help treat it, some sage would be good.

- *Memory loss.* There are quite a few herbs that could help treat this; Ginseng, purple sage, rosemary and ginko are some of the most effective.

- *Hardened arteries.* Cold feet and hands are the most common symptoms of this condition. Mistletoe, ginko and greater periwinkle are all good supplements to prevent this.

Other helpful herbs:

- *Gotu Kola for better mental performance and memory.* Also improves circulation to the brain.

- *Celery.* Restorative and prevents uric acid accumulation in the joins. Also improves circulation to the joints and muscles while detoxifying the blood.

- *Bladderwrack.* This seaweed variety is very rich in iodine and other minerals. It is also great for treating rheumatism and can be applied externally to the joints.

# Chapter 4: List Of Healing Foods

It is no secret that the food we eat directly affects our body and influences how it reacts. Some food products are great for you while others, even if they seemingly provide good benefits, actually do more damage. So, if you're trying to heal your body and remedy some issues that you might be having, making small changes in your diet just might be what you need. Here are a few great food items to consider adding to it:

— *Stress and anxiety*. Bananas are especially good for this purpose and you can have them however you want. Plain or with some yogurt, even with breakfast cereals.

— *Constipation and gas*. A cup and a half of live-culture yogurt would be your best remedy for this. Add some honey for a bit more flavor.

— *High blood pressure*. A handful or about sixty raisins contains about a gram of diber and 212 mg of potassium, both recommended for stopping hypertension.

— *Prevent kidney stones*. Eight dried apricots would contain 3mg of sodium, 2 gram of fiber and 325 mg of potassium, all of which are known for preventing mineral accumulation in the urine.

— *Stomach troubles and cramps*. Basil contains a compound called eugenol which is known to prevent both. It can kill of bacteria such as listeria and salmonella, which helps you avoid diarrhea as well.

— *High cholesterol*. Pears are a relatively underused fruit for this purpose. A medium sized one contains 5 grams of dietary fiber in the form of pectin which then flushes out bad cholesterol in the body.

- *Ulcers.* Cabbage contains sulforaphane, a potent compound which actually eliminates the H. pylori bacteria that causes peptic and gastric ulcers before it even enters your gut.

- *Fatigue.* There are some days wherein we can't avoid feeling fatigued. To get right back up on your feet, try freshly squeezed citrus juice. Orange would be the best for this as it can get rid of oxidative stress that's caused by free radicals. Just like with getting a shot of vitamin C, you'll feel instantly refreshed.

- *Yeast infection.* Garlic contains potent essential oils that can help resolve this health issue. You can take it however you want. In sauces, with your meats or even directly chew on raw pieces for maximum effect.

# Chapter 5: Using Essential Oils For Natural Cures

Besides food, there are also plenty of other natural resources that you can use to treat and cure anything that might be ailing you. Essential oils are direct byproducts of organic materials and they often contain the most potent compounds from the plant itself.

Here are a few essential oils that can be used as natural cures:

- *Lavender.* The most well-known essential oil has antiviral and antibacterial properties which can significant reduce the amount of time needed to heal stings, scrapes and bites.

- *Peppermint.* This one helps in alleviating heat due to fever. It can also help with motion sickness and nausea. Another great thing it can be used for is relieving the intensity of migraines or headaches.

- *Eucalyptus.* Often used as a vaporizer or inhaler, this helps in quickly relieving colds and coughs. It clears and disinfects the lungs and nasal passages, helping the patient to quickly recover. It is also antibacterial, antiviral and antispasmodic.

- *Tea tree oil.* Another potent antiseptic. This can be used on fungal infections, scrapes, warts, cuts, insect bites and even dandruff. It is most often used as an acne treatment.

- *Roman Chamomile.* Much gentler than tea-tree oil, it is a much better option for delicate skin when it comes to treating acne and acne scars. It can also be used on diaper rash and eczema.

- *Jasmine.* One of the most expensive oils, it is typically used to calm the mind and relax tense muscles. It is also known to enhance libido.

- *Lemongrass.* If you have infections, lemongrass is the safest way of treating it. It can also be used as an antiseptic and is a powerful antimicrobial oil so you can be sure that it would kill all the bacteria where you put it.

# Chapter 6: Why Natural Cures Vs. Traditional Medications

Still unconvinced about why you should switch things up and opt for natural cures instead of traditional medications? Here's a quick comparison of the two to help you understand better.

– Holistic

Traditional medicine will help treat your ailments but it can also affect other healthy parts of your body while doing so.

Natural remedies can treat your ailments just as well but without affecting other parts of your body negatively. In fact, it can even benefit it with continuous use.

– Gentleness

Traditional medicine can be quite harsh on the body considering it contains chemicals. This is why some patients often feel weak after taking them.

Natural remedies, on the other hand, are far gentler to the body. Because they're made out of organic ingredients, the same ones you eat, they will not make you feel weak.

– Side effects

Traditional medicine has plenty of side effects associated with it. In fact, you'll be warned about it when you read through the packaging or the instructions. Risks of these and risks of that; are you willing to give it a try?

Natural remedies would not have the same kinds of side effects. The only risks commonly associated with it are allergies and those are quite easy to avoid.

– Costs

Traditional medicine can be quite expensive because it takes a lot in order to produce and sell it. Of course, not everyone can afford the price but everyone will need them at some point.

Natural remedies are far cheaper to produce and even sell. You can even find some of them in your (or your neighbor's!) garden.

# Chapter 7: Natural Cures For Migraines And Headaches

Migraines and headaches are extremely common, almost everyone would experience them at some point during their life. The reason for it could vary greatly, from stress to simple weather changes. What remains the same is the remedy used for it. While manufactured meds work against them quite effectively, they do carry certain side effects that not everyone is keen on. Luckily, there are a number of all natural home remedies that you can use.

Below you'll find a list of the top home remedies for migraines and headaches:

– Cayenne

For this, you will need ¼ teaspoon of cayenne powder that's been diluted in 4 ounces of warm water. Take a clean cotton swab, wet it in the solution and dab some of it on the inside of your nostril. Once you start feeling the heat, it's a sign that it's working. It's uncomfortable at first but definitely effective.

– Feverfew

You'll need an ounce of fresh or dried flowers and a pint of boiling water. Steep for about ten minutes then strain. Drink this tea twice a day as needed.

– Apple cider vinegar

You'll need ¼ cup of apple cider vinegar mixed with about 3 cups of boiling water. On the side, keep a cup of cool water. This is for you to drink later on. Now, once the mixture begins to steam, place a towel over your head and hold your face over the bowl. Don't get too close because it might get hot. Inhale the steam for about 5 to 10 minutes or until it begins to cool down.

– Fish oil supplements

Take a tablespoon of quality fish oil and simply swallow it. Follow it up with some orange juice to get rid of the taste but if you're using a good brand, the taste shouldn't be a problem at all.

# Chapter 8: Natural Cures For Skin Diseases And Acne

For many teenagers and even adults, acne is a constant battle with one's skin. You wouldn't be the first one to try just about anything in order to get rid of it and gain back smoother, clearer skin. But maybe, that is where the problem lies. You're using one too many harsh chemicals on your face and not allowing it to breathe.

Why not go all natural with your skincare? It's risk free and won't cause damage to your skin at all.

Here are a few tips:

- Oil cleansing

Instead of a facial scrub or soap, try using an oil cleanser. With this, you'll be able to remove any dirt on your skin without damaging it. In fact, your face would feel much smoother after.

- Apple cider vinegar toner

There are plenty of uses for this particular kitchen condiment and among them would be for your face. Mix it with 1/3 of it with 2/3 of alcohol free witch hazel. It'll be the best for calming acne down.

- Honey and oats facial

If you don't have the time for the spa but need to gently exfoliate your skin, a mixture of honey and raw oats would be the best alternative. Keep it on your face for at least ten minutes before rinsing off with warm water.

- Tea tree oil spot treatment

Mix some of this with your preferred carrier oil and dab a bit on any acne you see. It will quickly dry it up and leave no scarring in its wake.

# Chapter 9: Natural Cures For Arthritis

Any person, regardless of age, could get arthritis. While there are different treatments available for it, nothing can beat going natural,especially if you're treating arthritis symptoms in younger kids as well as the elderly. For them, something gentle but effective is what's needed.

Shall we take a look at some of the best all-natural options?

– Aloe Vera

Well-known for its healing properties, you only need to externally apply this to any aching joints. A soothing massage using this would also be very helpful in relieving any pain or inflammation.

– Boswellia

Praised by many natural medicine practitioners for its potent anti-inflammatory properties, this is another plant that you can use for relieving arthritis. It is capable of blocking Leukotrienes which is the substance that attacks healthy joints, causing pain and inflammation.

– Turmeric

The same spice that you use for cooking curry also has anti-inflammatory properties which can help you in dealing with arthritis symptoms. Unlike the others, however, it is best taken orally. Not only can it ease joint pain, it is also capable of preventing rheumatoid arthritis progression.

– Willow Bark

This has been in use since the time of Hippocrates when patients were asked to chew on the bark to treat inflammatory infections. Today, the same can still be done but most people prefer it in tea form. Do note that having the right amount is crucial because too much of it can cause mild irritations.

– Thunder God Vine

One of the oldest herbs used for medicine, the extract from its skinned roots can be applied and massaged directly onto the area to relieve pain.

# Chapter 10: Natural Cures For High Blood Pressure

When it comes to high blood pressure, there are many different pills and supplements that are supposed to help you keep it in check. However, many of these can also be quite harsh on the body, with some even becoming the cause of liver damage and early onset of deafness. Surely you want none of that, right?

Try some of these natural remedies for high blood pressure. They work just as effectively but without the added side effects.

- Cinnamon

A favoriteof many, this particular seasoning can effectively lower blood pressure in people who have diabetes. The best bit is that you can easily add it to any dish or even drink!

- Cardamom

Another popular seasoning, it is known to have a number of health benefits and among them, lowering high blood pressure. For the effects to manifest, however, they need to be taken everyday. So add the spice to your stews, soups and even baked goods.

- Garlic.

This one is no secret. It has the ability to lower your blood pressure significantly by making your blood vessels dilate and relax. In doing so, the blood is then able to flow freely hence lowering pressure. Take it everyday by adding it fresh to your favorite dishes. You can also ingest it in supplement form.

- Celery Seed

Often used to flavor soups and other savory dishes, it also carries with it the ability to effectively treat hypertension. In fact, Chinese traditional medicine has been using it for centuries for this purpose. You can choose to juice the entire plant or use the seeds for flavoring, it has the same effect.

    –   French Lavender

Though not commonly used as a culinary herb because of its perfumed smell, its flowers can be added to baked goods. It is effective for lowering blood pressure.

# Conclusion

Thank you again for purchasing this book on *Natural Cures: 20 Natural Cures, Herbal Medicines, And Natural Remedies For Increased Overall Health And Beauty!*

I am extremely excited to pass this information along to you, and I am so happy that you now have read and can hopefully implement these strategies going forward.

I hope this book was able to help you understand the benefits of natural remedies and how to use them for yourself. The next step is to get started using this information and to hopefully live a healthier and more natural life!

Please don't be someone who just reads this information and doesn't apply it, the strategies in this book will only benefit you if you use them! If you know of anyone else that could benefit from the information presented here please inform them of this book.

Finally, if you enjoyed this book and feel it has added value to your life in any way, please take the time to share your thoughts and post a review on Amazon. It'd be greatly appreciated!

Thank you and good luck!

# Preview Of:

## *Incredible Herbal Remedies!*

# <u>Herbal Remedies</u>

## *Herbs, Spices, And Oils To Cure Common Ailments, Prevent Sickness, Improve Health And Fight Disease!*

# Introduction

I want to thank you and congratulate you for purchasing the book, *"Herbal Remedies: Incredible Herbal Remedies! - Herbs, Spices, And Oils To Cure Common Ailments, Prevent Sickness, Improve Health And Fight Disease!"*

This "Herbal Remedies" book contains proven steps and strategies on how to:

- Benefit from affordable, safer and effective treatments for common ailments, chronic conditions and diseases using herbal remedies;

- Prevent sickness with herbs, spices and essential oils;

- Use the healing powers of herbs, spices and oils to improve your health;

- Do oil pulling to stop and prevent tooth decay, gum problems and improve your oral health;

- Use herbs as your natural anti-aging solution so you don't have to spend much for costly skin care products;

- Use honey for medicinal purposes;

- Use apple cider vinegar for weight loss;

- Start sustainable gardening of herbal plants.

These and more are yours to enjoy when you start reading the contents of this book. Use this book as your guide to benefit from one of Mother Nature's greatest gifts to humanity - incredible herbal remedies.

Why entrust your life entirely on pharmaceutical medicines when you can benefit from herbal remedies for health conditions that do not necessitate medical intervention?

Thanks again for purchasing this book. I hope you enjoy it!

# Chapter 1: 4 Incredible Things Herbal Remedies Can Do

Herbal remedies continue to increase in popularity. More and more people choose to benefit from these natural remedies to treat their ailments and protect their health. In fact, the World Health Organization (WHO) approximates that about 80% of the entire world population include herbal medicines as part of their health treatment.

In this chapter, you will discover four (4) of the incredible things that herbal remedies can do. You may have not yet known about some of these things and your physician may never tell you about the other things.

More Affordable Treatment

Using herbs as natural remedies enables you to save your hard-earned money. Saving money may not be possible with pharmaceutical medicines given their typically high cost. Aside from being the more affordable solution for ailments, botanical remedies are also equally effective compared to drug-based medications.

The Harvard Medical School recognizes the ability of botanicals to heal. In fact, it has published a special health report on how to treat common pain conditions without using drugs or surgery. Results from several studies and research likewise show that plant-based medications work well with the body systems.

Safer Treatment than Drugs

Herbs and other natural remedies are safer treatment than drug-based medicines. Typically, herbal medicines do not carry side effects because of their natural composition. Drugs, on the other hand, contain active ingredients that interfere with the body systems; hence, the side effects.

Side effects of pharmaceutical medicines often occur (a) when you start taking the medication, (b) change the dosage either to lower it or to strengthen it and (c) when you stop taking your medicine(s). In contrast, the side effects that may happen with herbal treatments are normally attributable to the improper use of the medication.

Potency Similar to Pharmaceuticals

At first glance, herbal medicines may not be as potent as pharmaceutical medicines when it comes to comparing their dosage. For instance, a cup of tea of willow bark (naturally containing aspirin and works as a pain reliever) is weaker in dosage than the standard dosage of pharmaceutical aspirin.

However, instead of looking at the dosage comparison, look at the effects of these medications. If taking a cup of willow bark can suffice to relieve your pain, why risk your general health to the typical side effects of pharmaceutical medicines? Keep in mind a general rule in medication: start taking your medicine with the lowest dosage possible.

More Effective Treatment for Chronic Conditions

Unless your medical condition needs urgent intervention or treatment, herbal remedies are usually more effective than drug-based medications. With chronic conditions, treatment may require a longer period involving repeated use of the medication(s). This could mean greater risks of side effects with pharmaceuticals.

Botanicals, on the other hand, have no side effects or minimal side effects only. As mentioned earlier, the side effects typically occur only with improper use or dosage. Herbs contain natural chemicals that can sufficiently address chronic health conditions without the risk of side effects.

## Thanks For Previewing My Exciting Book Entitled:

## "Herbal Remedies:Incredible Herbal Remedies! Herbs, Spices, And Oils To Cure Common Ailments, Prevent Sickness, Improve Health And Fight Diseases!"

To purchase this book, simply go to the Amazon Kindle store and simply search:

"HERBAL REMEDIES"

Then just scroll down until you see my book. You will know it is mine because you will see my name "Sarah Brooks" underneath thetitle.

Alternatively, you can visit my author page on Amazon to see this book and other work I have done. Thanks so much, and please don't forget your free bonuses

**DON'T LEAVE YET! - CHECK OUT YOUR FREE BONUSES BELOW!**

# Free Bonus Offer: Get Free Access To The www.LuxyLifeNaturals.com VIP Newsletter!

Once you enter your email address you will immediately get free access to this awesome newsletter!

But wait, right now if you join now for free you will also get free access the "Secrets of Becoming A Meditation Expert – In 7 Days!" free Ebook!

To claim both your FREE VIP NEWSLETTER MEMBERSHIP and your FREE BONUS Ebook on the SECRETS OF BECOMING A MEDITATION EXPERT IN 7 DAYS!

Just Go To:

# www.LuxyLifeNaturals.com